THE ULTIMATES CIALIS GUIDE

A Modern Guide to Enhancing Performance, Confidence, and Connection Naturally

Marco Albrecht

Copyright © 2025 by [Marco Albrecht]

All rights reserved. No part of this publication may be reproduced, stored in a retrieval system, or transmitted in any form or by any means—electronic, mechanical, photocopying, recording, or otherwise—without the prior written permission of the author, except for brief quotations used in a review or scholarly work.

This book is intended for informational purposes only and is not a substitute for professional medical advice, diagnosis, or treatment. Always consult your physician or qualified health provider with any questions you may have regarding a medical condition.

The author and publisher disclaim any liability for any adverse effects resulting directly or indirectly from the use or application of the information contained in this book.

Disclaimer

This book is for informational and educational purposes only. It is not intended to replace medical advice, diagnosis, or treatment from a qualified healthcare provider. Always speak with your doctor or healthcare professional before starting or changing any medication, supplement, or treatment plan.

The author has made every effort to ensure the information in this guide is accurate and up to date at the time of publication, but medicine and health advice may evolve over time. The reader assumes full responsibility for how they choose to use this information.

Every person's body and situation is unique—what works for one individual may not work for another. This book is meant to inform and support, not to prescribe or guarantee specific results.

Table of Contents

Chapter 1: Understanding Cialis—What It Really Is 5
   Introduction 5

Chapter 2: The Benefits of Cialis Beyond the Bedroom 7
   Improving Blood Flow and Circulation 7

Chapter 3: When and How to Take Cialis 12

Chapter 4: Common Side Effects and How to Handle Them 16
   Mild Side Effects: Headaches, Flushing, and More 16

Chapter 5: The Role of Nutrition in Sexual Health 22

Chapter 6: Confidence, Connection, and Communication 26
   How Performance Affects Self-Esteem 26

Chapter 7: Cialis and Relationships—What You Both Need to Know 31
   Setting Expectations Together 31

Chapter 8: Special Considerations for Men at Different Life Stages 36
   Cialis in Your 30s, 40s, 50s, and Beyond 36

Chapter 9: When Cialis Isn't Enough—What to Do Next 42
   Evaluating Underlying Causes of ED 42

Chapter 10: Creating Your Personal Performance Plan 48
   Setting Realistic Goals for Sexual Wellness 48
   The end 53

Chapter 1: Understanding Cialis—What It Really Is

Introduction

Cialis is the brand name for the medication **tadalafil**, a prescription drug approved by the U.S. Food and Drug Administration (FDA) to treat erectile dysfunction (ED), benign prostatic hyperplasia (BPH), or both. It belongs to a group of drugs known as **PDE5 inhibitors** (more on that soon).

Unlike older ED treatments, Cialis offers unique benefits that have helped millions of men regain confidence and control. One of its biggest advantages? **Its long-lasting effect**—up to 36 hours in some cases. That's why it's often nicknamed "the weekend pill."

But Cialis isn't just about erections—it's about options. You can take it **daily at a low dose** or **as needed at a higher dose**. This flexibility makes it easier to match your lifestyle and relationship needs.

In short, Cialis is a modern, versatile treatment designed to support your sexual health without interrupting your life.

How Cialis Works in the Body

To understand how Cialis works, it helps to know a bit about how erections happen. When a man becomes sexually aroused, signals from the brain and nerves cause blood vessels in the penis to relax. This relaxation allows more blood to flow in, creating an erection.

An enzyme called **PDE5 (phosphodiesterase type 5)** can sometimes interfere with this process by narrowing blood vessels too quickly or preventing them from fully expanding. This is where Cialis comes in.

Cialis **blocks the action of PDE5**, allowing the blood vessels in the penis to stay relaxed longer. This leads to increased blood flow, which helps produce and maintain a firm erection when you're sexually stimulated.

Key Differences

- **Longer Duration**: Cialis outlasts all others, which means more flexibility and less pressure to "time things perfectly."

- **Daily Use Option**: Cialis is the only one approved for daily dosing, allowing for more spontaneous intimacy.

- **Food Interaction**: Cialis is less affected by food than Viagra or Levitra, which means you don't have to skip your meal.

Each medication has its pros and cons. Some men prefer the shorter window of action from Viagra or Levitra, while others value the freedom Cialis provides. It's all about finding what fits your needs and lifestyle.

Chapter 2: The Benefits of Cialis Beyond the Bedroom

Improving Blood Flow and Circulation

One of the most important ways Cialis works is by **improving blood flow**. While this is essential for sexual function, better circulation can support other aspects of health too.

How Cialis Helps

Cialis is part of a class of medications called **PDE5 inhibitors**, which help relax and open up blood vessels. This leads to **increased blood flow**, especially in the pelvic region. While this helps with erections, it also supports better **vascular health** in general.

Improved blood circulation may benefit:

- **Heart and vascular system health** (though Cialis is not a treatment for heart disease)
- **Leg and pelvic blood flow**, which can help reduce discomfort from poor circulation
- **Exercise performance**, for some individuals with certain medical conditions

While Cialis is not approved as a heart medication, the way it improves blood flow can have a **positive side effect** on how you feel during physical activity.

Important Note: Always consult your doctor before using Cialis if you have any heart-related conditions. It is not a substitute for heart medication or lifestyle changes.

Supporting Confidence and Mental Well-Being

Erectile dysfunction is more than a physical issue. It often affects how you feel about yourself, your confidence, and even your emotional connection with your partner. The ability to perform sexually can impact **self-esteem, mood, and mental health** in powerful ways.

The Confidence Loop

When you're confident in your body's ability to respond, your anxiety about sexual activity decreases. This reduces stress, which in turn makes it easier to perform. This is often called the **confidence loop**, and Cialis can help jumpstart it.

Many men report that once they started using Cialis:

- They felt more in control
- They began to look forward to intimacy again
- Their performance anxiety dropped
- They experienced improved communication with their partner

Cialis, by helping the physical aspect of erections, can also indirectly support **emotional healing** and **mental clarity**.

Cialis for Benign Prostatic Hyperplasia (BPH)

You may be surprised to learn that Cialis is also **FDA-approved to treat symptoms of benign prostatic hyperplasia (BPH)**. BPH is a non-cancerous enlargement of the prostate that affects many men, especially as they age.

Common BPH Symptoms:

- Frequent need to urinate (especially at night)
- Difficulty starting urination
- Weak urine stream
- Incomplete bladder emptying
- Feeling like you always need to go

These symptoms can significantly affect quality of life. Cialis helps by **relaxing the muscles in the prostate and bladder**, which makes it easier to urinate and reduces urgency.

This means that **Cialis isn't just for ED**. If you're dealing with both ED and BPH, it might be a two-in-one solution that simplifies your treatment plan and improves daily comfort.

Long-Term vs. As-Needed Use

Cialis comes in two forms:

1. **Daily Use (2.5 mg or 5 mg)**
2. **As-Needed Use (10 mg or 20 mg)**

Each option has its own advantages, depending on your goals and preferences.

Daily Use Benefits:

- Helps with both ED and BPH
- Allows for **spontaneity** in sexual activity
- Provides steady levels of the drug in your system
- Reduces performance pressure or anxiety
- Becomes part of your **regular routine**, like taking vitamins

As-Needed Use Benefits:

- Ideal for **occasional** intimacy
- Less medication overall
- Flexibility to use when you choose

- Works within **30 to 60 minutes**

Some men even start with as-needed use and switch to daily dosing if they want more consistency or are also managing BPH symptoms.

Tip: Talk to your healthcare provider about which dosing schedule matches your health needs, lifestyle, and relationship preferences.

Emotional and Relationship Benefits

Sexual health isn't just about the body—it's about connection, communication, and closeness. When intimacy suffers, relationships often feel strained. Many couples struggle to talk about ED, leading to misunderstandings and emotional distance.

How Cialis Helps Rebuild Connection

By supporting a man's ability to perform sexually, Cialis can help couples:

- **Reconnect physically and emotionally**
- **Build trust** through shared experiences and vulnerability
- **Reduce resentment or confusion** that may have built up over time
- **Strengthen communication** about sexual needs and desires

Cialis offers an opportunity for couples to **rebuild intimacy** together. When the physical barriers are lowered, emotional healing often follows.

Many men also report that Cialis helps them feel **more in tune with their partner's needs**—not just sexually, but emotionally. That's a powerful shift in any relationship.

Additional Well-Being Considerations

Cialis isn't a replacement for healthy habits, but when used alongside good nutrition, exercise, and stress management, it can support an overall sense of **vitality and well-being**.

Combined with Lifestyle Changes:

- **Exercise** improves natural blood flow and testosterone levels
- **Balanced diet** supports cardiovascular and prostate health
- **Stress reduction** helps reduce performance anxiety and tension
- **Sleep** improves hormone regulation and energy levels

Chapter 3: When and How to Take Cialis

Taking Cialis correctly is key to its effectiveness. It's a medication that works with your body—not instantly, but when the timing and context are right.

For Daily Use:

- Take it at the **same time every day**, with or without food.
- Try to make it part of your daily routine, like brushing your teeth or taking vitamins.
- Consistency matters. It may take **4 to 5 days** for the medication to reach full effectiveness in your system.

For As-Needed Use:

- Take it **30 to 60 minutes** before sexual activity.
- It can be taken **with or without food**, but avoid heavy or high-fat meals close to the time you take the pill.
- Only one dose should be taken in a 24-hour period.

Cialis does **not cause an automatic erection**. Sexual stimulation is still required for it to work.

Tip: Plan ahead but stay relaxed. The medication gives you a window of opportunity—not a strict schedule.

How Long It Lasts and What to Expect

One of Cialis's biggest advantages is how long it lasts. While other ED medications may wear off after a few hours, Cialis can remain effective for up to **36 hours** in many men.

What That Means for You:

- You don't have to rush into sex

- You can try again later if things don't go as planned

- It allows for a more **natural and less pressured** experience

What You May Feel:

- You may notice increased firmness during arousal

- Erections may feel more consistent or easier to achieve

- You may feel more confident initiating intimacy

Every man's body responds differently. Some men notice results quickly; others may need a few tries to find the best dosage and timing.

If Cialis doesn't work the first time, don't give up. It may take **several attempts**, especially if stress or anxiety is a factor.

Timing Around Food, Alcohol, and Other Medications

Food

- Cialis can be taken with or without food.

- However, **high-fat meals** may slightly delay how fast it works.

- For best results, avoid heavy meals right before taking as-needed doses.

Alcohol

While moderate alcohol (one or two drinks) is generally safe, **too much alcohol can increase the risk of side effects** and reduce the effectiveness of Cialis.

Heavy drinking while using Cialis can cause:

- Low blood pressure

- Dizziness or fainting

- Headaches or flushing

If you plan to drink, keep it **moderate and balanced with food**.

Other Medications

Cialis can interact with certain drugs, especially:

- **Nitrates** (used for chest pain): These can cause a dangerous drop in blood pressure when combined with Cialis.

- **Alpha-blockers** (used for prostate or blood pressure issues): Can also cause blood pressure issues.

- **Antifungals or antibiotics**: Some may increase Cialis levels in your body.

Always tell your doctor about all medications, supplements, or herbs you're using—even over-the-counter ones.

Tips for Maximizing Results

To get the best outcome from Cialis, a few practical tips can make a big difference.

1. Set the Right Expectations

Cialis enhances your body's ability to have an erection when sexually stimulated. It does not increase sexual desire or act like an aphrodisiac. Relax and allow the medication to support you—not carry the entire weight of the moment.

2. Communicate With Your Partner

Let your partner know you're using Cialis. This can help reduce pressure, increase understanding, and open up emotional intimacy. You may even find that the conversation itself brings you closer.

3. Manage Stress and Performance Anxiety

Worrying too much about performance can reduce the effectiveness of Cialis. Try deep breathing, mindfulness, or light exercise beforehand to relax your body and mind.

4. Maintain Healthy Habits

Good health supports better results. Regular exercise, a balanced diet, and sufficient sleep all help with blood flow and hormone balance. If you smoke, consider quitting—it can interfere with circulation and reduce the effects of Cialis.

5. Work With Your Doctor

If you're not getting the results you want, don't be discouraged. Dosage adjustments, timing changes, or switching from as-needed to daily use may help. Your doctor can guide you through these options safely.

Chapter 4: Common Side Effects and How to Handle Them

Mild Side Effects: Headaches, Flushing, and More

Most people who take Cialis either don't notice any side effects or only experience mild ones. These effects often fade as your body adjusts to the medication. Here are the most common ones:

1. Headache

This is the most frequently reported side effect.

Why it happens:

Cialis improves blood flow by relaxing blood vessels. This can temporarily widen blood vessels in the head, leading to mild to moderate headaches.

How to handle it:

- Drink plenty of water
- Avoid alcohol and caffeine, which can make it worse
- Use over-the-counter pain relievers like acetaminophen (if approved by your doctor)

2. Facial Flushing

You may notice a warm feeling or redness in your face or neck.

Why it happens:

This is caused by increased blood flow near the skin's surface.

How to handle it:

- Stay cool—flushing often fades on its own
- Avoid spicy foods, alcohol, or hot drinks around the time you take your dose

3. Nasal Congestion

You might feel a bit "stuffy" after taking Cialis.

How to handle it:

- Try breathing steam or using a saline nasal spray
- Decongestants may help but ask your doctor first, especially if you have high blood pressure

4. Indigestion or Stomach Discomfort

Also known as dyspepsia, this may feel like bloating or mild heartburn.

How to handle it:

- Eat smaller, lighter meals
- Avoid greasy or spicy foods
- Use antacids only if approved by your healthcare provider

5. Muscle Aches and Back Pain

These side effects can appear 12 to 24 hours after taking Cialis and usually go away within two days.

How to handle it:

- Stay hydrated and stretch gently
- Use heat or cold packs on sore areas
- Ask your doctor about over-the-counter pain relief

6. Dizziness or Lightheadedness

A drop in blood pressure can cause dizziness in some users.

How to handle it:

- Sit or lie down if you feel faint
- Stand up slowly from a seated or lying position
- Avoid alcohol and stay hydrated

Serious Side Effects to Watch For

While most people tolerate Cialis well, some rare side effects can be serious. It's important to recognize these symptoms and know when to seek help.

1. Chest Pain or Pressure

Cialis should never be used with **nitrate medications**. If you have chest pain while using Cialis, get medical help right away.

2. Sudden Vision Changes

This includes blurry vision or sudden loss of sight in one or both eyes, especially in people with eye conditions or risk factors like high blood pressure or diabetes.

What to do:

Stop using Cialis and seek emergency medical attention.

3. Sudden Hearing Loss

Though rare, some users have reported a sudden decrease or loss of hearing, sometimes with ringing in the ears (tinnitus) or dizziness.

What to do:

Stop the medication and contact a doctor immediately.

4. Allergic Reactions

Signs may include rash, itching, swelling, or difficulty breathing.

What to do:

Get emergency help. This could indicate a serious allergic reaction.

5. Prolonged or Painful Erections

Known as priapism, this condition involves an erection lasting more than four hours. If untreated, it can cause permanent damage.

What to do:

Go to the emergency room right away if this happens.

How to Minimize Discomfort

Managing side effects often starts with **how and when you take Cialis**. Here are simple strategies to improve your experience:

1. Start with the Lowest Effective Dose

If you're sensitive to medications or new to Cialis, talk to your doctor about starting at a lower dose and adjusting as needed.

2. Take it With Food (If Needed)

While Cialis works with or without food, a small meal can sometimes reduce side effects like stomach upset.

3. Stay Hydrated

Water helps flush the medication through your system and can ease headaches and muscle aches.

4. Avoid Alcohol

Alcohol can make certain side effects worse—especially flushing, headaches, and dizziness. If you drink, do so in moderation.

5. Stick to a Consistent Routine

Taking Cialis at the same time each day (if using daily) can help your body adjust and reduce surprises.

Managing Cialis Alongside Other Health Conditions

If you have other medical conditions, it's especially important to use Cialis wisely. Talk openly with your doctor so your treatment plan is safe and effective.

Conditions to Discuss Before Using Cialis:

- **Heart disease or recent heart attack**
- **Stroke history**
- **Liver or kidney problems**
- **Low or high blood pressure**
- **Eye problems like retinitis pigmentosa**
- **Blood cell disorders like sickle cell anemia**
- **Stomach ulcers or bleeding issues**

Medications to Mention:

- **Nitrates** for chest pain
- **Alpha-blockers** for prostate or blood pressure issues
- **Antifungals and antibiotics**
- **Seizure or HIV medications**

Even herbal supplements can interact with Cialis, so share your full list of remedies—even over-the-counter products.

Tip: Bring a written list of all your medications to doctor appointments. This helps avoid dangerous interactions.

Chapter 5: The Role of Nutrition in Sexual Health

What you eat directly affects your circulation, hormone levels, and energy—all of which influence sexual performance.

1. Eat More Heart-Healthy Foods

Cialis works by improving blood flow. A healthy heart and flexible blood vessels make it even more effective.

Include:

- Leafy greens (spinach, kale)
- Berries (blueberries, strawberries)
- Fatty fish (salmon, mackerel)
- Nuts (walnuts, almonds)
- Whole grains (brown rice, oats)

These foods support nitric oxide production, reduce inflammation, and help lower blood pressure.

2. Limit Processed and High-Sugar Foods

Sugary snacks, fried foods, and processed meats can stiffen arteries, increase belly fat, and raise insulin resistance—all of which reduce Cialis's impact.

3. Stay Hydrated

Dehydration can cause fatigue and affect blood volume. Drinking enough water supports circulation and energy levels.

4. Maintain a Healthy Weight

Excess body fat, especially around the abdomen, is linked to lower testosterone and poor blood flow. A modest weight loss can significantly improve erectile function.

Exercise and Circulation

Physical activity is one of the most effective ways to naturally improve sexual function and enhance Cialis's effectiveness.

1. Aerobic Exercise

Cardio exercises like walking, jogging, swimming, or cycling improve heart health and blood flow. Aim for at least 30 minutes, five days a week.

2. Strength Training

Lifting weights or doing bodyweight exercises supports testosterone production and helps regulate blood sugar.

3. Kegel Exercises

These target the pelvic floor muscles and can improve erection strength and control. Contract the muscles used to stop urination, hold for five seconds, and repeat 10–15 times.

4. Stay Consistent

Regular movement keeps blood vessels flexible, reduces stress, and supports energy levels—all essential for sexual health.

Supplements That May Help

While supplements aren't a substitute for healthy habits or medication, some may support sexual health when used responsibly.

1. L-Arginine

An amino acid that helps the body produce nitric oxide, improving blood flow. It may work synergistically with Cialis but should only be used under medical guidance.

2. Ginseng (Panax)

Known as a traditional remedy for improving libido and performance. It may help boost energy and reduce stress.

3. Zinc

Essential for testosterone production and sperm health. Deficiency can lower libido.

4. Maca Root

An adaptogen that may support mood, stamina, and sexual desire.

Important: Always talk to your doctor before combining supplements with Cialis. Some interactions could be harmful or reduce the drug's effectiveness.

Managing Stress and Anxiety

Even with Cialis, psychological factors like stress and anxiety can interfere with sexual performance. Your mind and body are deeply connected.

1. Practice Deep Breathing

Slow, mindful breathing reduces heart rate and calms the nervous system. Try inhaling for 4 seconds, holding for 4, and exhaling for 6.

2. Meditation and Mindfulness

Daily mindfulness practice has been shown to reduce performance anxiety and improve confidence.

3. Talk It Out

Whether it's a partner or a therapist, sharing your thoughts and concerns can relieve tension and build emotional intimacy.

4. Get Enough Sleep

Lack of sleep affects hormone levels and mood. Aim for 7–9 hours of restful sleep each night.

Lifestyle Habits That Support Sexual Vitality

1. Avoid Smoking

Smoking damages blood vessels and decreases nitric oxide availability, directly impairing erection quality.

2. Limit Alcohol

While a drink or two may help you relax, too much alcohol reduces testosterone and affects nerve sensitivity.

3. Stay Connected

A supportive, connected relationship promotes emotional safety—which enhances arousal and desire.

4. Routine Health Checkups

Conditions like high blood pressure, diabetes, or hormonal imbalances often go unnoticed. Regular checkups help keep your body in balance.

5. Focus on Pleasure, Not Just Performance

Sometimes focusing only on the goal of an erection increases pressure and stress. Exploring intimacy in a relaxed and open way can actually improve sexual function.

Chapter 6: Confidence, Connection, and Communication

How Performance Affects Self-Esteem

Erectile dysfunction is not just a physical issue—it can deeply impact how a man sees himself. When performance suffers, it's easy to internalize that as a reflection of one's worth, masculinity, or desirability.

The Emotional Impact of ED

Many men feel:

- Embarrassed or ashamed
- Anxious about future sexual encounters
- Fearful of rejection or disappointing their partner
- A sense of "losing their edge" or manhood

These feelings are valid—and common. But it's important to remember that ED is a **medical condition**, not a personal failing. Just like high blood pressure or diabetes, it can be managed with the right approach.

Reframing Your Identity

Cialis can restore function, but true confidence goes beyond performance. Confidence comes from:

- Accepting yourself
- Being honest about your needs
- Knowing you're more than just your physical ability

It's okay to feel vulnerable. In fact, owning your experience and choosing to take action is a sign of strength, not weakness.

Communicating With Your Partner

ED and intimacy challenges don't just affect you—they affect your relationship. But silence can create confusion and distance. Talking openly with your partner about what you're experiencing is one of the most healing steps you can take.

Why Honest Communication Matters

When you hide what's going on, your partner may:

- Assume you're no longer attracted to them
- Think the issue is emotional or personal
- Feel confused, rejected, or hurt

By being open, you help your partner understand that:

- ED is medical, not emotional
- You're seeking solutions (like Cialis)
- You care about the connection and want to work together

How to Start the Conversation

It's normal to feel nervous, but honesty builds trust. Try saying:

- "I've been struggling with performance lately, and I want you to know it's not about you."
- "This has been difficult for me, but I want to be open so we can face it together."
- "I'm taking steps to improve things, and I hope we can talk about it openly."

You don't need to have all the answers. Just starting the conversation shows courage and builds emotional intimacy.

Rebuilding Emotional Intimacy

Sex isn't just about physical performance—it's about connection, vulnerability, and emotional closeness. For many couples, the journey to overcoming ED can actually strengthen the bond between them.

Intimacy Beyond Intercourse

Sometimes, the pressure to perform creates anxiety that gets in the way of pleasure. Exploring other ways of being intimate—without the goal of penetration—can remove that pressure and increase enjoyment.

Examples include:

- Touching, cuddling, or massage
- Deep conversations
- Shared experiences (like taking a walk or trying a new activity together)

Slow Things Down

Cialis gives you the opportunity to regain spontaneity, especially with daily use. Use this flexibility to slow down, focus on connection, and enjoy the moment. The goal is not just an erection—it's feeling present, connected, and emotionally close.

Healthy Masculinity and Sexual Identity

Cultural messages about masculinity often make men feel like they must always be strong, virile, and in control. When ED enters the picture, it can challenge these ideas and lead to shame or withdrawal.

Redefining Strength

True strength is not about never struggling—it's about how you respond when challenges arise. Taking care of your health, asking for help, and seeking emotional connection are all marks of maturity and confidence.

Sexuality Is a Journey

Your sexual identity isn't tied to one specific function or moment—it evolves over time. You can still be a passionate, loving, and confident man even if you face performance challenges. Cialis can support your physical side, but embracing your full self—emotional, intellectual, spiritual—brings true power to your relationships.

The Role of Trust and Vulnerability

Trust is the foundation of a strong relationship. When you're facing sexual challenges, building or rebuilding trust with your partner helps both of you feel safe and supported.

What Is Vulnerability?

Vulnerability means being open about your fears, emotions, and needs. It's not weakness—it's a doorway to deeper love.

When you share your experience with ED:

- You create space for empathy
- Your partner can respond with care and support
- You become allies, not adversaries

Building Trust Over Time

Trust grows through:

- Consistency: showing up, being present
- Honesty: sharing feelings without blame

- Patience: understanding that healing takes time

Chapter 7: Cialis and Relationships—What You Both Need to Know

Setting Expectations Together

What Cialis Can and Can't Do

Cialis (tadalafil) is a highly effective medication that improves blood flow to support erectile function. But it's important for both partners to understand that it's not a "magic switch."

Cialis:

- Helps achieve and maintain an erection when arousal is present
- Doesn't automatically create desire or arousal
- May take time to work effectively (depending on the type and dosage)
- Can be affected by factors like stress, fatigue, or relationship tension

Setting expectations together means understanding that while Cialis can help with the physical aspect of ED, rebuilding trust and intimacy is a process. Progress may be gradual.

Being Patient with the Process

It can take time to find the right dosage, timing, and rhythm that works for you. Being patient with each other helps reduce pressure and promotes a relaxed, supportive environment. Celebrate small wins, and remember: intimacy is about connection, not perfection.

Discussing ED Openly and Respectfully

Why Communication Matters

ED can bring up uncomfortable feelings—shame, guilt, frustration, even resentment. If left unspoken, these emotions can create distance between partners. Honest, respectful communication creates space for healing and growth.

How to Start the Conversation

If you're the one experiencing ED:

- Choose a calm, private time to talk
- Use "I" statements (e.g., "I've been feeling anxious about intimacy lately")
- Be honest about what you're experiencing and how it's affecting you

If you're the partner:

- Listen without judgment
- Express care and support
- Avoid blaming or taking the situation personally

Common Phrases That Help

- "This isn't about attraction or desire—it's something physical we're working on."
- "You're not alone. I want to support you."
- "Let's figure this out together."

Creating a Safe Space

Respect means honoring each other's emotions without trying to "fix" everything. Sometimes just being heard is enough. Keep the focus on teamwork, not blame.

Restoring Connection and Enjoyment

Rebuilding Intimacy Beyond Performance

When ED has been present, physical closeness may have been avoided out of fear or embarrassment. Cialis can help restore function, but emotional closeness and comfort take effort too.

Try rebuilding intimacy in gradual, low-pressure ways:

- Cuddling, touching, or holding hands
- Non-sexual physical affection
- Talking about fantasies, memories, or what feels good emotionally and physically
- Sharing laughter and positive experiences

Reducing Performance Pressure

Taking the focus off "performance" and putting it on shared enjoyment can ease anxiety. Consider saying:

- "Let's just be close without expectations."
- "It's not about what happens next—I just want to enjoy being with you."

Creating space for playfulness and exploration can reduce tension and deepen intimacy.

Being Emotionally Present

True connection comes from emotional presence. That means being attentive, affectionate, and open—even when things don't go perfectly. Vulnerability can actually strengthen your bond.

Supporting Your Partner's Needs

For the Partner of Someone Using Cialis

ED can affect you too. You may have your own feelings: sadness, rejection, confusion, or fear. That's normal. Supporting your partner doesn't mean ignoring your own needs.

Talk openly about what you need emotionally and physically. A supportive relationship includes mutual care.

Encourage Without Pressure

Support your partner without pushing:

- Be encouraging, not demanding
- Celebrate progress, not perfection
- Let them know you appreciate their efforts

Show Affection Consistently

Affection isn't just sexual. Small gestures—a touch, a compliment, a kind word—can help your partner feel seen and valued, even outside the bedroom.

Creating a Shared Plan for Intimacy

Make Intimacy a Team Effort

Rather than seeing ED as "his" issue or Cialis as a solo solution, create a shared plan that supports both of you. This can include:

- Talking about when and how to use Cialis (e.g., planned vs. daily use)
- Exploring what kind of touch or intimacy feels good
- Setting the tone for relaxation and connection (e.g., planning date nights, turning off distractions)

Keep the Conversation Going

Sexual health evolves. What works one week might not work the next. Keep checking in with each other about what feels good, what's working, and what you both need.

Focus on the Relationship

Use this opportunity to reconnect in other areas of your relationship:

- Improve emotional closeness
- Share new experiences together
- Work on shared goals outside of the bedroom

Chapter 8: Special Considerations for Men at Different Life Stages

Cialis in Your 30s, 40s, 50s, and Beyond

In Your 30s: Stress, Lifestyle, and Early Signs

If you're in your 30s and starting to notice difficulties with erections, it can be frustrating—and even surprising. At this stage, ED is often less about aging and more about factors like:

- High stress levels
- Anxiety around performance
- Poor sleep
- Alcohol, smoking, or recreational drug use
- Beginning signs of health conditions (like high blood pressure)

Cialis can be helpful in boosting blood flow and reducing performance anxiety by giving you more time and flexibility. However, it's just as important to explore lifestyle adjustments that support long-term function.

Tip: Use this decade as a wake-up call. Take any changes seriously and work with a healthcare provider to identify root causes, rather than just relying on a pill.

In Your 40s: Hormonal and Metabolic Shifts

In your 40s, testosterone may start to decline gradually. You might notice changes in energy, libido, or muscle mass. This is also when blood pressure, cholesterol, and blood sugar levels may begin to shift.

Cialis may become more helpful during this stage, especially for men who:

- Experience occasional erectile issues
- Have early signs of cardiovascular changes

- Need more flexibility in sexual timing (e.g., weekend doses or daily low-dose Cialis)

At this age, it's important to think of Cialis as one part of a bigger plan—including managing weight, reducing stress, and checking hormone levels.

Tip: Ask your doctor about testing your testosterone levels if your libido or energy feels off. Sometimes hormonal support alongside Cialis makes a big difference.

In Your 50s: Managing Physical and Emotional Transitions

By the time you reach your 50s, you may be juggling work stress, health concerns, and changes in relationship dynamics. Erectile issues can become more common—not just because of aging, but because of:

- Slower circulation
- Side effects of medications (like those for blood pressure or cholesterol)
- Emotional disconnect or relationship stress
- Lower testosterone

This is a good time to talk with your doctor about the best way to use Cialis. Daily dosing may help keep you ready and reduce anxiety, while the as-needed version may still work well for some.

Tip: Make intimacy a regular part of life, not just a "special occasion." Planning regular connection can actually improve performance and satisfaction over time.

In Your 60s and Beyond: Maintaining Vitality

Sexual activity in your 60s, 70s, or later can be just as satisfying—though it often requires a more thoughtful approach. At this stage, men may be managing:

- Chronic illnesses (like diabetes or heart disease)

- Prostate issues
- Reduced sensation or slower response to arousal
- Physical fatigue

Cialis has been shown to work well for older men, especially when used consistently. But safety becomes a bigger priority, especially with other medications or health conditions.

Tip: You don't have to give up a satisfying sex life. Focus on pleasure, connection, and emotional intimacy—not just performance.

Managing Age-Related Changes

Circulation and Blood Flow

Healthy erections require healthy blood vessels. As you age, arteries can stiffen, and blood flow may slow. Cialis helps by relaxing blood vessel walls, but its effectiveness can be limited if underlying vascular health is poor.

What Helps:

- Regular aerobic exercise
- Managing blood pressure and cholesterol
- Quitting smoking
- Staying hydrated

Hormones and Libido

Testosterone levels drop about 1% per year after your 30s. That doesn't always mean you'll need hormone therapy—but if you notice low sex drive, fatigue, or mood changes, it's worth checking.

What Helps:

- Strength training
- Quality sleep
- Healthy fats (avocados, nuts, olive oil)
- Stress reduction

Medication Side Effects

As men age, they're more likely to be on medications that can impact sexual function—like antidepressants, beta-blockers, or diuretics. Cialis may still work, but dosage and interactions need to be considered.

What Helps:

- Talk to your doctor before combining medications
- Keep a list of all prescriptions and supplements
- Monitor any new symptoms that arise

Heart Health and Cialis Use

One of the most important considerations at any age is how Cialis affects your heart—and vice versa.

Cialis and the Cardiovascular System

Cialis increases blood flow, which means it works in part on your circulatory system. For men with stable heart disease, Cialis is generally safe. But there are important precautions:

Do NOT use Cialis if:

- You take nitrates (e.g., nitroglycerin)
- You have unstable angina or very low blood pressure

Cialis may help:

- Improve exercise tolerance in men with mild heart failure
- Lower blood pressure slightly (especially with daily use)

Talk to Your Cardiologist

If you have a history of heart problems, always clear Cialis use with your cardiologist. Many men mistakenly think they have to give up sex after a heart event—when in fact, restoring intimacy can boost mental and physical health.

Tip: If you can climb two flights of stairs without chest pain, your heart can likely handle sexual activity. But always check with your doctor.

Talking With Your Doctor About Long-Term Plans

Cialis can be part of a long-term approach to sexual health, but it's not meant to be used in isolation from the rest of your health care.

What to Discuss With Your Doctor

- Your age and stage of life
- Your goals for intimacy and sexual performance
- Other medications and conditions
- Hormone levels and lab work
- Whether daily or as-needed use is right for you

Don't be afraid to bring it up—even if your doctor doesn't. Sexual health is an important part of quality of life.

Renewing Prescriptions and Monitoring Health

If you plan to use Cialis over many years, your doctor may want to:

- Check your blood pressure and heart rate
- Review kidney and liver function
- Reevaluate dosage and frequency annually

Tip: Keep a journal of how Cialis is working for you—what dosage you're using, when you take it, and how it affects your mood, energy, and performance.

Staying Sexually Active as You Age

Redefining What Intimacy Means

Sex doesn't have to look the same at every age. What matters is that it's satisfying and meaningful to you and your partner.

As you age, you might:

- Take more time for foreplay and connection
- Enjoy different positions for comfort
- Focus more on emotional closeness than performance

Keeping the Spark Alive

- Schedule time for intimacy—spontaneity can be harder with age
- Try new things—massage, sensual touch, or changing settings
- Use humor to ease anxiety and build connection

Staying Confident

Aging can challenge your body image, energy levels, and self-esteem. But sexual confidence isn't just about performance—it's about how you feel in your skin, how you connect with your partner, and how you embrace change with grace.

Chapter 9: When Cialis Isn't Enough—What to Do Next

Evaluating Underlying Causes of ED

Before jumping to new treatments, it's important to understand *why* Cialis may not be working as expected. ED is a symptom—often pointing to other areas of the body or mind that need attention.

Common Physical Causes

Even when using Cialis, physical barriers can limit its effectiveness. These include:

- **Vascular issues:** Poor blood flow due to clogged arteries or high blood pressure

- **Diabetes:** Nerve and blood vessel damage from long-term high blood sugar

- **Low testosterone:** Hormone imbalances that affect libido and energy

- **Obesity:** Inflammation, poor circulation, and reduced testosterone

- **Sleep apnea:** Poor oxygen levels during sleep can disrupt sexual function

A full medical check-up—including blood work, blood pressure, and hormone testing—can reveal if a deeper health issue is contributing to your ED.

Tip: Ask your doctor for a full physical and metabolic screening if Cialis isn't producing consistent results.

Emotional and Psychological Factors

Mental health plays a powerful role in sexual performance. Even if the body is capable, the brain has to be on board.

Common psychological causes include:

- **Performance anxiety**

- **Depression**

- **Stress from work or relationships**
- **Past trauma**
- **Low self-esteem**

These issues can block arousal and override the physical effects of Cialis. In some cases, anxiety about taking Cialis itself can lead to a self-defeating cycle.

Tip: If you find yourself overthinking during intimacy or worrying about "failing," the issue may be more emotional than physical.

When to Consider Therapy or Counseling

There's no shame in seeking emotional or relationship support. In fact, therapy can often succeed where medication alone cannot. Erectile dysfunction isn't just about getting an erection—it's about connection, confidence, and feeling desired.

Individual Therapy

Therapy can help uncover and address hidden stressors, past experiences, or self-image issues that may be affecting your sexual performance. Therapists trained in sexual health or cognitive behavioral therapy (CBT) can help you:

- Reduce performance anxiety
- Improve body image
- Manage depression or anxiety
- Rebuild self-confidence

Couples Counseling

If ED has affected your relationship, couples therapy can be incredibly healing. It's a safe space to talk openly, rebuild trust, and reconnect emotionally and physically.

- Improve communication around sex and intimacy
- Navigate frustrations or misunderstandings
- Build intimacy beyond just sexual activity

Tip: Therapy isn't just for crisis—it's a tool for growth. Even a few sessions can open the door to new levels of connection.

Exploring Combination Therapies

When Cialis works *partially* but not completely, combination therapy may be the answer. This means using Cialis alongside another method to improve results.

Cialis + Testosterone Replacement

If low testosterone is part of the problem, testosterone therapy (TRT) can improve libido, energy, and erectile response. Combined with Cialis, the results can be much more satisfying.

- Testosterone can be delivered via injections, gels, or patches
- Regular monitoring is essential to avoid side effects

Caution: TRT isn't right for everyone. Always get hormone testing and talk with your doctor first.

Cialis + Lifestyle Changes

Sometimes, improving health multiplies the effectiveness of Cialis. This includes:

- **Exercise:** Increases circulation, testosterone, and stamina
- **Diet:** Supports vascular health and hormone balance
- **Weight loss:** Improves blood flow and reduces ED severity
- **Sleep:** Restores hormone balance and improves mood

This "lifestyle combo" is especially powerful when combined with either daily or as-needed Cialis.

Cialis + Other Medications

If Cialis isn't working well on its own, your doctor may suggest trying another PDE5 inhibitor (like Viagra or Levitra) or adding a different type of treatment altogether.

Advanced Medical Options

For some men, especially those with long-term or severe ED, other medical treatments may be necessary. These options are safe and effective when used under the care of a qualified provider.

Vacuum Erection Devices (VED)

Also known as penis pumps, these devices draw blood into the penis using vacuum pressure. They're often paired with a tension ring to maintain the erection.

- Effective for many men with poor circulation
- Drug-free and relatively low-risk
- May take time to get used to

Penile Injections

These involve injecting a medication (like alprostadil) directly into the base of the penis. It sounds intimidating, but many men report high satisfaction.

- Quick and reliable
- Can be used when oral meds fail
- Requires training and proper dosing

Intraurethral Therapy

A small pellet of medication is inserted into the urethra using a special applicator. This delivers blood flow-enhancing medication directly to the tissue.

- Fast-acting
- Less invasive than injections
- May be less effective for some men

Penile Implants (Surgery)

For severe or long-term ED that hasn't responded to other treatments, a penile implant may be the best option.

- Surgically placed device inside the penis
- Allows for on-demand erections
- High satisfaction rates in appropriate candidates

    Tip: Surgery is a last resort—but it's life-changing for some men. Explore all options first, and work with a specialist who can guide you through the process.

Building a Supportive Care Team

You don't have to face ED alone—and you shouldn't. A collaborative care team can help you feel seen, supported, and empowered.

Who Should Be On Your Team?

- **Primary Care Provider:** For initial screenings and overall health
- **Urologist:** A specialist in male sexual and urinary health
- **Endocrinologist:** For hormone-related issues like low testosterone
- **Cardiologist:** If you have blood pressure or heart concerns

- **Therapist or Counselor:** For emotional and relationship support
- **Partner (if applicable):** Open communication with your partner can turn frustration into partnership

How to Advocate for Yourself

Many men suffer in silence because they feel embarrassed or dismissed. You have every right to seek answers and push for solutions that work for you.

- Write down your questions before appointments
- Track your symptoms and responses to treatment
- Be honest about what's working and what's not
- Don't give up if the first treatment doesn't work

Tip: ED is a health condition—no different than managing blood pressure or joint pain. You deserve compassionate care.

Chapter 10: Creating Your Personal Performance Plan

Setting Realistic Goals for Sexual Wellness

What Does "Success" Look Like to You?

Before you can create a performance plan, it helps to get clear on your own vision of success. Ask yourself:

- What does a satisfying sex life mean to me?
- What do I want more of—confidence, pleasure, connection, spontaneity?
- How do I want to feel before, during, and after intimacy?

There's no one-size-fits-all answer. For some men, the goal is achieving reliable erections. For others, it's feeling more emotionally present, reducing anxiety, or strengthening their relationship. Define your own version of wellness so you can build toward something meaningful.

Start Small and Build Gradually

Setting big goals is exciting—but success usually comes from taking small, consistent steps. For example:

- Start with using Cialis on weekends or during planned moments.
- Add light exercise to improve circulation.
- Introduce new habits one at a time (e.g., cutting back on alcohol, improving sleep, trying mindfulness).

Your personal performance plan should feel achievable and positive—not overwhelming or strict. Think progress, not perfection.

Tracking What Works for You

Why Self-Tracking Matters

Tracking your experiences helps you learn what works—and what doesn't. It also helps reduce anxiety by replacing guesswork with patterns and insight. You don't have to write a daily report, but a few simple notes can go a long way.

What You Might Track

- **When you take Cialis:** time of day, dosage, with or without food
- **Effectiveness:** how well it worked, how long it lasted, side effects (if any)
- **Mood and stress levels:** your mental and emotional state before intimacy
- **Lifestyle habits:** sleep, exercise, alcohol, or food that may have influenced outcomes
- **Relationship dynamics:** how connected or supported you felt with your partner

Over time, you'll begin to notice trends. Maybe you feel best when you take Cialis after a good night's sleep. Maybe stressful workdays impact performance. These insights help you adjust your plan based on real-life feedback.

Combining Medical and Natural Approaches

Why a Holistic Plan Works Best

Cialis is powerful—but it works best when paired with healthy habits. Combining medical treatment with natural strategies creates synergy. Each part supports the others.

Core Areas to Focus On

1. **Nutrition**
   A diet rich in whole foods, lean protein, healthy fats, and plenty of fruits and vegetables helps improve blood flow, hormone levels, and energy. Limit excess sugar, alcohol, and processed foods.

2. **Exercise**

   Regular movement supports cardiovascular health, testosterone production, and mental well-being. Even walking daily can make a noticeable difference. Aim for a mix of aerobic and strength-building activity.

3. **Sleep**

   Good sleep supports everything from sexual function to hormone regulation. Poor sleep can blunt Cialis's effects and reduce libido. Prioritize 7–9 hours of quality rest.

4. **Stress Management**

   Chronic stress raises cortisol, disrupts focus, and impairs arousal. Try breathing exercises, meditation, nature walks, or therapy—whatever helps you decompress and stay present.

5. **Supplements (if needed)**

   Some natural supplements may support sexual health when used responsibly. These might include L-arginine, zinc, maca root, or ashwagandha. Always consult your healthcare provider first.

6. **Emotional Health**

   ED often carries emotional weight—shame, fear, or doubt. Addressing these feelings (with your partner or a professional) can ease anxiety and boost confidence.

By combining the physical benefits of Cialis with these healthy lifestyle choices, you create a strong foundation for sexual wellness that lasts.

Staying Consistent Without Obsession

The Power of Consistency

Consistency is key to making real change—but it doesn't mean being perfect. The goal is to stay on track most of the time, without being rigid or self-critical. Think of your performance plan as a flexible routine, not a strict rulebook.

- **Build habits gradually:** Add one new habit every week or two.
- **Stack habits:** Link new routines to existing ones (e.g., stretching after brushing your teeth).
- **Celebrate small wins:** Progress isn't always about big breakthroughs. A night of good sleep or a relaxing, pressure-free date counts too.

Avoid Over-Focusing on Results

It's easy to get caught up in outcome thinking—did I get an erection? Did everything go perfectly? But focusing too much on results can increase pressure and decrease enjoyment.

Instead:

- Focus on connection over perfection.
- Allow space for learning and adjustment.
- Recognize the value of simply showing up for yourself and your partner.

Remember: Your sexual wellness is a journey. Treat yourself with the same patience and encouragement you'd offer a close friend.

Living With Confidence, Passion, and Purpose

More Than Just Performance

While sexual performance is one aspect of wellness, the ultimate goal is a fulfilling, confident life. Your personal performance plan can support broader goals: better health, deeper relationships, greater self-respect.

Confidence doesn't come from never failing—it comes from continuing to show up and grow. Each time you take a step forward, you're building momentum and resilience.

Connecting With Your Partner

Don't forget the importance of shared intimacy. Invite your partner into the conversation. Ask:

- What do you enjoy most about our time together?
- How can we support each other better?
- What would make intimacy more meaningful or fun?

Creating shared goals helps deepen your bond and turns challenges into opportunities for growth together.

Keeping the Big Picture in Mind

Sexual health is part of your overall life story. As you get older, your needs and goals will evolve—and that's natural. The habits and insights you build now will continue to serve you in every area of life.

You deserve to feel strong, desired, and fully alive—both in and out of the bedroom.

The end

Made in United States
North Haven, CT
17 July 2025